Feelings Explained: Emotions Tamed

Understanding the Inner Messages Behind Your Emotions

Chris W.E. Johnson

Feelings Explained: Emotions Tamed
Understanding the Inner Messages Behind Your Emotions

Chris W.E. Johnson

[1]

Contents

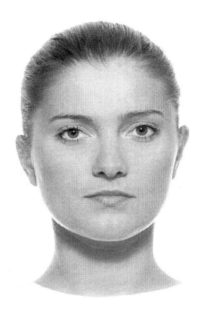

[3]

Introduction and Intent

People in the Mind/Body/Spirit movement often proclaim the New Age mantra, *You Create Your Own Reality*. But what does this really mean? And how exactly, as the metaphysical literature would have us believe, do we create *everything* in our personal reality—including the unpleasant things such as an illness or an accident? Furthermore, surely the reality of a hoodlum snatching my new phone and running off with it has nothing to do with my own creative abilities!

Seth, a metaphysical character channeled by *the Seth material* (see *References and Resources*) author Jane Roberts between the 1960s and 1980s, first coined the expression. Careful study of the Seth material (now housed at the Yale University Library and regarded by transpersonal psychologists as *the* leading metaphysical source), reveals exactly what *"you create your own reality"** means, and crucially, *how* we go about creating our reality—our personal reality and our collective, co-created reality—including the realities we wish we hadn't created.

[4]

Since the 1990s, perhaps due to the approach of the worrying times we now live in, a growing number of channelling psychics have come to the fore. Abraham (through Esther Hicks), Bashar (Darryl Anka), Elias (Mary Ennis), and Omni (John L. Payne), are but a few *"energy personality essences"* relaying valuable information on how we go about forming our realities. Reassurance is on offer to those of us frightened by the realities of these fraught yet highly significant times of dissolution, degradation, and downfall.

My *It's About You!* trilogy brings together a wide variety of teachings on how we create our *personal* reality. Book I, *Know Your Self*, explores material provided by numerous metaphysical, philosophical, spiritual, and scientific sources—synthesizing profound knowledge on the true nature of our physical reality into a consistent, clear message.

Reality creation: The primary ingredients

What you perceive to be your reality is the result of a complex mix of psychical energies which includes the thoughts, beliefs, feelings and emotions that your *personality** attracts, grows, and allows to flow through it. Of these psychological elements, your *beliefs* hold the key to what you eventually manifest in the physical realm. They form a psychological membrane, a sieve through which you sift the energies of your thoughts, feelings and emotions before you bake them into the cake of your reality. This book focuses on how *feelings* and *emotions* become involved in the process of baking your reality.

The primary intent of this book is to help you realize the difference between the energies of your

[5]

feelings and emotions so that you can consciously understand and utilize both. Its aim is to bring clarity on what a feeling or emotion is telling you about your current situation and how to then go about addressing any negative feelings and/or emotions.

Our shift in consciousness

Our shared, co-created physical reality is a manifestation arising from the predominant beliefs held within the collective psyche of humankind. It is the ultimate cake of a myriad layers and flavors baked in a psychic oven as vast as the sun. As you are doubtless aware, there is a great deal of change happening in our co-created reality. Political, sociological, religious and ecological changes abound and the first half of the 21st Century will see a radical overhaul of these and other, what are essentially, *belief systems.**

The *intent** of *human consciousness*—to know our "Self" and place within *Consciousness** and to fully express our magnificent capabilities—drives this change in our collective psyche. This evolutionary psychical development is now commonly referred to in the Body/Mind/Spirit movement as our *shift in consciousness.**

A fundamental psychical outcome for humanity in this shift is that we come to realize and appreciate how our beliefs, along with our thoughts, feelings, and emotions, construct our realities. Beliefs are the blueprints in the manifestation process and negative emotions guide us to the beliefs we have that need attention. Seth informs us:

[6]

The nature of your personal beliefs in a large measure directs the kinds of emotions you will have at any given time. You will feel aggressive, happy, despairing, or determined according to events that happen to you, your beliefs about yourself in relation to them, and your ideas of who and what you are.

(Roberts, J. (1974) *The Nature of Personal Reality: A Seth Book.* Englewood Cliffs, NJ: Prentice-Hall Inc. p. 230.)

The Difference Between Feelings and Emotions

First, one thing needs to be perfectly clear.

Feelings are *different* **from emotions. You can have a feeling without there being an emotion present, but an emotion is always preceded by a feeling.**

They do have one thing in common however—both are independent electromagnetic energy forms that help you express yourself in the physical world. Their energies are neither positive nor negative as we are wont to describe them— it's our *conscious-mind** that labels them as such.

Crucially, most feelings function as a mechanism for *initiating* **action, whereas emotions are a potential energy resource for** *concerted* **action.**

Feelings are an integral part of how your physical self functions. Emotions, on the other hand, maintain an existence in the *electric field** and are not a part of your physical expression unless "invited" (by your psychological disposition) to be so. As with thoughts, emotions do not require a host mind to exist and you can choose to entertain them or not.

Feelings alert the conscious-mind to information or knowledge about to transfer directly from your *inner self** and/or *body-consciousness**. In short, **feelings are a signalling mechanism.** The transfer may seem instantaneous, or when the signal is of the *emotional-signal** variety, a momentary delay occurs for purposes of conscious acknowledgement. We are yet

[8]

to understand the significance of the delay, although according to **Elias** (see *References and Resources*), it is a crucial moment of choice between *re*-**acting** to the impending information or taking more considered action.

Emotions are not signalling mechanisms. They gain conscious awareness through the preceding emotional-signal, as they usually, not always, enter processing through the *solar plexus chakra route**. Feelings are very often a stimulus to act, with the emotional-signal type of feeling informing you of emotional energy held in readiness should you do so.

We constantly equate the *feeling* of an emotional-signal with the emotional energy that we most often *unconsciously* allow to flow into our physical systems. Consequently, we believe such signals to be the same as emotions, thereby confusing the two differing forms of energy and distorting or misinterpreting the information contained within them.

Feelings associate with the body-consciousness, emotions with the personality

Another factor that distinguishes feelings from emotions is the way in which your inner self handles them. Your inner self will only send feelings to your conscious-mind after it has consulted the body-consciousness. This is because **the layer of the Self that *feels* feelings and generates a high proportion of them is the body-consciousness.** Your inner self and body-consciousness work in harmony to offer the conscious-mind the *information* contained within feelings and *the strength of any feeling* indicates the level of importance your inner self puts upon the information in transmission.

[9]

Emotions on the other hand, belong to the personality. They are the connective forces that bind your spiritual (inner) self to your physical self. Therefore, your inner self will work with your personality when dealing with emotional energy.

The personality is the portion of the Self that manages and channels emotional resources. It is responsible for holding emotional energy from immediate release and does so under instruction from the inner self—usually with a regard for overall health. It will also hold emotional energy when instructed by the *ego-self**—often delusive instruction formulated from fearful beliefs, or by way of coping with a traumatic event.

If your personality holds an emotion's energy to it, it does so for a reason. Any subsequent release of this energy becomes a *significant event* as the emotional energy has gained *important psychological meaning.* This meaning changes the emotion from its pure energy form to an energy form *with a communication.*

The strength of any emotion, following an emotional-signal type of feeling, indicates the level of importance your inner self assigns to the *psychological communication* carried by the emotion.

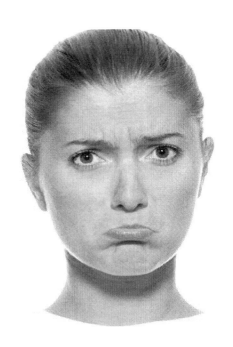

[11]

Feelings

Most feelings are to do with relaying information to the conscious-mind as instantaneously as possible. An experience that virtually all of us have enjoyed that illustrates the immediacy of feelings is feeling inspired. When we think about it, inspiration is an experience that often puzzles us—in the sense that we wonder where the idea came from that accompanies the feeling. We may assign it to an active imagination, but we will intuitively know that it came from our inner self *to inspire us* along our life's intentional path.

Although the body-consciousness can itself generate a feeling and relay it immediately to the conscious-mind (think of the feeling of coldness one might get when entering an empty room), the inner self is almost always collaborating with the body-consciousness when instigating the feeling of pain—whether psychological, emotional, or physical in nature. Physical pain is of course a direct communication to the conscious-mind that we should act immediately.

An enduring physical pain, along with emotional and psychological pain, communicates that your beliefs need serious review and adjustment.

Many of us dismiss feelings (even painful ones) as unimportant, even though we constantly receive numerous kinds of feeling signals. They come as sensations through the *throat chakra**; a sense of awareness of our internal state (emotional-signal) through the solar plexus chakra; and feelings akin to intuition, but more profound, signalling a direct awareness of the vitality of *Divine Love,** through the *base chakra**. We can also throw *impulses** and *impressions** into the mix of energy forms that vie for attention in our conscious-minds.

Please note that if you ignore a negative feeling it is likely to persist, escalate in intensity, and eventually become mentally, emotionally, or physically debilitating.

Dealing with a "negative" feeling when in conversation

If you sense a negative feeling when talking with someone, it can mean either your *Essence self** is sensing that their *feeling-tone** does not resonate with yours (see feeling-tone in Glossary of Terms)—or your inner self and body-consciousness have teamed-up to produce an emotional-signal. An emotional-signal implies that you are allowing his or her negativity (their expressed thoughts and beliefs) to grow in your mind.

Know that a negative emotional-signal is asking you to act in one of two ways.

The first way is simply to accept that their expression has a detrimental effect on how you feel in the moment, so don't allow his or her ideas to concentrate in your mind and disassociate yourself from the conversation. If the feeling is overwhelmingly oppressive, either end the conversation or just change the subject.

[13]

Trust in this feeling and appreciate that each person chooses the thoughts they wish to share, albeit usually without conscious awareness of the feelings they can generate in others. Your inner self is essentially asking you to use *your* conscious awareness of the feeling-tone or emotional signal. It wants you to maintain good feelings about your Self, so choose whether to accept the thoughts and ideas on offer, or to politely end the conversation.

Furthermore, it's not your job to insist that others accept your own thoughts and ideas because they make *you* feel good. Trust and appreciate that the thoughts you are offering in return produce a positive effect on you, but others are free to take them or leave them. You do not need to defend that which makes you feel good. If you find yourself doing this, then know that you are denigrating your inner self by not trusting in its guidance — **good feelings are indications from your inner self that you are in tune with who you are and your** *personal intent**. As **Bashar** (see *References and Resources*) points out:

The only reason anyone would force someone into their point of view, is because they don't [inwardly] believe in their point of view.

The second way to respond to a negative emotional-signal is to explore it. If the feeling has roused an emotion, then know that your inner self is asking you to examine your beliefs. You don't need to begin a belief examination immediately you sense an emotional charge, just appreciate the *fundamental* message (take a look at your beliefs here), and resolve to investigate it when you next have a quiet moment for yourself.

[14]

Remember that your *Garden of Beliefs** contains *all* beliefs, but not all thoughts. Perhaps you need to realize that the negative thoughts another person offers are already growing in your garden into a belief and you are unaware of this, or you are denying it.

See where the feeling takes you. Is the person expressing thoughts that generate an emotional-signal that has an emotional charge attached? Are you sensing anger, hate, guilt, jealousy, envy, or any other negative emotion? If so, and you find yourself rising to the emotion, perhaps embracing it, or finding it difficult to dismiss, then you have an awareness of a belief within you that requires attention. **Remember:**

Feelings, followed by emotions, shadow your beliefs.

Or, as **Bashar** puts it,

There is no such thing as a feeling without a point of view [belief] that creates the feeling.

Work with the feel of your feelings

According to Elias, it is important to us from an evolutionary perspective to begin recognizing and interpreting the variety of feelings we experience as they originate from the nonphysical or spiritual aspects to our Self (body-consciousness, Essence, or inner self)—which means they always contain information or instruction for our physical self's benefit and expansion.

We can begin this expansion by listening to and trusting our inner self's guidance mechanisms—feelings, impressions, and impulses. This in turn will move us into trusting our Self and letting go of fear.

[15]

We're used to working with the outer sense of touch and distinguishing between the feel of various physical surfaces. Essential to any personal shift in consciousness is to become used to working with our *inner senses** and discerning between the *feel* of our feelings.

We lazily sort the nuances of our feelings into either good or bad sensations. We then don't fully appreciate the good ones in case they might be sinful, and don't investigate the bad ones because we're scared to go there. **Ironically, bad feelings are *good***—in the sense that they have the potential to teach us more about our Selves and the reasons as to *why* we don't feel so good!

Important inner-information speaks to us through the signals of our feelings and the voice of our emotions. You can count on the fact that if the information is not important, we wouldn't get the feeling. If it wasn't *especially important*, it wouldn't have emotional energy backing it.

By attaching information to an uncomfortable feeling, your inner self is suggesting that before your conscious-mind can come to a considered response, it needs to check with your personality for any emotional involvement. If present, the emotion's intensity reflects how imperative it is that you attend to your beliefs. An emotion can *scream* at you at times. It does so because it is in your Garden of Beliefs that you will find the reasons behind any form of negativity you are experiencing.

You will find the reasons hidden amongst the roots of your beliefs. Uncovering them may require some digging but bringing them into the light of awareness can substantially alter

[16]

the landscape and thus the disposition of your personality. Seth reminds us:

> You will not understand your emotions unless you know your beliefs. It will seem to you that you feel aggressive or upset without reason, or that your feelings sweep down upon you without cause if you do not learn to listen to the beliefs within your own conscious mind, for they generate their own emotions.
>
> (Roberts, J. (1974) *The Nature of Personal Reality: A Seth Book.* Englewood Cliffs, NJ: Prentice-Hall Inc. p. 230.)

Emotions

Emotions are an element of your expression that you have chosen to be the method, so to speak, of your expression within this particular physical dimension. This is not to say that other physical dimensions do not incorporate emotion, for some do, but within this particular dimension, it is one of the base elements of your creation of expression. *(Elias.)*

Emotions always come with a communication. They are born as a subjective communication to an objective awareness—a message from your spiritual self to your physical self's conscious-mind. Your personality, in collusion with your inner self, instigates the communication. Within any situation, if an emotional-signal feeling invokes an emotional response that carries a negative tone (anxiety, anger, sadness, guilt, anything that makes you feel bad), the communication's essential point is that you carefully consider your actions, if not in the moment, then as soon after acting as possible.

Information encapsulated within a negative emotion provides the most precise documentation of what you are creating in the moment and how the creation interferes with your overall intent. It is therefore important for you to acknowledge and examine the entirety of the communication. Conversely, it's just as important to heed and appreciate *positive* emotions as they are indicative of your manifestations being in alignment with your desires and intent.

[18]

Our tendency is to focus simply on the tone of the emotional-signal and then assume that any accompanying emotion gives us license, as well as the energy, to *react* to the situation in a manner befitting the initial signal. If we sense anger rising within us, for example, we are likely to act in an aggressive way. Our actions focus on the emotional-signal of anger and the following emotion's energy drives our actions along while we remain in total ignorance of the message contained within.

Whether negative or positive in nature, emotional-signal feelings can consume a lot of energy, particularly if we perpetuate them. Ignoring them can perpetuate them, or we can use the energy of an associated emotion to keep the feeling of an emotional-signal going—**as happens when we** *worry.* Because they can consume a great deal of energy, thus potentially draining the body's physical systems to a point of exhaustion, the body-consciousness will automatically subdue such feelings when need be. The conscious-mind interprets these automatic interventions as the ebb and flow of feelings.

An intervening body-consciousness offers some reprieve from negative feelings and its subduing actions also explain why positive feelings don't hang around either. Being in a constant state of excitement for example—now often referred to as being *hyperactive*—is also of course a drain on energy resources.

If you sense that negative feelings are beginning to perpetuate, then **Abraham's** (see *References and Resources*) suggestion that you deal with them as soon as you can by turning your thoughts to more positive ones is well worth considering.

Omni (see *References and Resources*) reminds us that, "Emotions are the result of thought; they don't spring up without there being a sponsoring thought."

By refocusing your thoughts, you *consciously* help your body-consciousness with its energy management. If emotional energy has taken the feeling to an intensity that makes it difficult for you to change your thoughts, you can employ some "tapping" (see *What To Do About The 3Ds*), but then you must, when calmer, pay attention to the emotion's communication and act upon it. Such diligence will then make it unnecessary for your inner self, personality, and body-consciousness to generate this emotional-signal again!

Positive or negative?

We regard emotions as either positive or negative in tone—joy is a positive emotion to experience, whereas anxiety is clearly negative. Our channelled guides use this positive/negative contrast to simplify things. Essentially, they are saying that positive emotions (when you're feeling good)—such as joy—come with the message that you (your physical self) are *at this moment* in vibrational alignment with the personal intent and purpose for this lifetime set by your Essence self. You are allowing the energy to flow through you unimpeded by any fears and in tune with the vitality of Divine Love.

Negative emotions (when you feel bad)—such as anxiety—inform you that you are presently out of vibrational alignment with your Essence self's ambitions, off the path of your life's purpose, and in need of some serious quality time to meditate on what ails you.

Getting angry?

The emotion of anger, as an example, contains the message that your conscious-mind is finding its choices on how to act in the current situation severely restricted. What's restricting its choices? The answer is a *firmly held belief.*

Anger can begin with the emotional-signal of frustration—which is telling you that you are *beginning* to shut down your freedom of choice—beginning to stimulate the energy behind the firmly held belief. As emotional energy rises within you to the point of anger, you are imagining your choices are becoming increasingly confined—until rage takes over and you are only able to perceive one possible choice of action.

There are always choices available to you in *any* **situation.** Yes, anger provides you with plenty of energy to physically respond to the situation, but it is also telling you that you have certain beliefs that are restraining your choice of response. The *intensity* of emotion tells you that the belief is at the *core* of your thinking as it *demands* that you respond in a habitual manner—no matter whether any actions taken are inappropriate to the current circumstances, or more significantly, are violent in nature.

What to do

As with any negative emotion like anger, you need (for optimum psychological health) to act on one fundamental therapeutic principle—**examine your beliefs and modify them as soon as possible.**

With anger, your inner self asks you to identify and examine the belief that is generating your thoughts in the current moment. Simply becoming aware of the belief that's affecting you begins the therapeutic process. After an angry interlude, when you're calm, just ask yourself the question, "What is the predominant belief that I associate with this situation? And do I regard it to be absolutely *true*?" Bashar tells us:

You cannot have an emotion without believing something to be true.

There are very few absolute truths. Truths, you see, are usually *core beliefs** that have grown—*through the investment of a great deal of energy*—to the status within your mind of a "truth." Being human is really all about managing our thoughts, beliefs, feelings and emotions. And we can always *choose* and *change* what we believe. Even if we believe a core belief to be true!

So, if the *truth* of the matter is that the Earth is obviously flat as your physical senses show it to be, then realise you can modify this **belief** to something like: I currently *believe* that the Earth is spherical, as shown by the scientific instruments that extend our physical senses such as telescopes.

Love and fear are not really emotions

What we think of as the primary emotions, love and fear, are more accurately to do with our *state of being** (see *Glossary of Terms)*. This is a psychological *state* that sits on a continuum, with feeling "*love*-ly" (in tune with our Essence) on one end, a

[22]

"neutral" state somewhere in the middle (navigating the circumstances with no great emotional involvement), and fear at the other end (arrived at through the pattern of our thoughts and beliefs about the circumstances).

Fear has a complexity of "layers" — from the beneficial impulse (remember, impulses are feelings, not emotions) to act immediately when in danger — to a fundamentally debilitating state of mind that has your inner self issue a communication — attached to a fear-based emotion — that you are generating a lack of trust within yourself.

This is usually to do with a lack of trust in your *creational* abilities, but ask yourself, "What is it about the situation that stimulates a distrust in my ability to respond consciously, rather than resort to an impulsive fight or flight response? What is it that I believe to be true about myself that can generate this fearful emotion?"

The bottom line is that fear tells you that you *don't* hold the belief that you can create your own reality.

To genuinely believe that you create your own reality is of course scary in itself — it would mean that you are *responsible* for everything that occurs in your life. Frightening perhaps, but then this energy can just as easily be channelled into excitement!

Whether we believe it or not

According to our metaphysical friends, Seth in particular, whether we believe it or not, *"you create your own reality"* is an inescapable truth that pertains to what we perceive to be "real" — that is, made physical within the objective, physical plane of our existence. It is one of those very few truths, facts or

[23]

principles that apply to our *physical* existence within Consciousness.

We will come to realize that emotions are the life force of this physical plane, as they are integral to its expression *through* our Selves. It is because we are currently unfamiliar with the dual role of emotions—energy *and* communication—that we remain in abject confusion as to their true nature and importance to our well-being. Until we fully understand them, we will continue to habitually react to certain situations rather than respond to them in a fully informed, objective, and self-developing manner. It is important to remember that it's not the emotion that has you *re*-act; it's the situation that triggers a controlling, reactionary belief.

An emotion is not a reaction to the circumstances; it is informing you of all the factors that go into creating the circumstances. *(Elias.)*

Once we recognize that emotions are an energy resource with a message from our inner self, our freedom of choice of action opens. An emotional event brings to our attention the subtler details of the experience.

For this reason, when your thoughts appear to be in chaos, turn your attention to what you are creating in the moment. Do you sense negative emotion involved in the creation? If so, know that it contains vital information about *why* you've created the experience, information worthy of investigation if not in the moment, then when you are able.

Most of us assume that we have little control over our emotions. Emotions appear to be forces outside of us—

independent organisms akin to viruses and bacteria whose energies will help us either resolve a situation or make matters worse. Emotions *are independent forms of energy*—that is, they do not come attached to a belief (we do the attaching in our minds)—so a belief is not required for their expression.

However, they are very much a part of the human expression, intimately interwoven into our psychological structuring and our ability to express ourselves in the physical domain. As Seth reminds us, they are the *life force* of this dimension of existence we call physical reality. We have a lot more to learn about emotions as **they are key to the creation of our reality.**

The Inner Messages Behind
Your Emotions

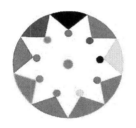

Feelings and emotions have different communicational intent. One alerts the conscious-mind to subconscious information or knowledge, the other arises because of a belief we hold to be "true."

A special type of feeling signals the imminent arrival of an emotion that provides both energy for action and valuable information concerning, amongst other things, our psychological constructs. I call this special feeling an *emotional-signal*, as its aim is to alert the conscious-mind to not only energy waiting in the wings, but also to energy already being held behind a core belief.

An emotional-signal is triggered when the current physical and mental circumstances are causing the held energy, and thus belief, to take automatic control over our actions.

Imagine you're feeling angry. The emotional-signal feeling is essentially telling you that, in this type of situation, you are not in full conscious control. Lack of conscious control can easily result in violent actions causing harm to yourself or others. Furthermore, the emotional energy in waiting, if not fully utilized or released (*productively*) in the moment, will likely add energy to that already stored and further entrench the core belief as a "truth." This in turn will lead to less and less conscious control over one's actions in similar circumstances.

Remember that our physical self, energy body and mind, are designed to allow energy to flow through us into physical manifestation. Impeding or holding energy within the physical self frustrates the full expression of our personality.

[28]

One thing we need to remember when dealing with a "negative" emotion is to be mindful of the information it contains and act upon it. Presently, we tend only to administer to the emotional-signal that *precedes* the emotion—which may bring temporary relief from the following emotion's effects but will not normally provide a permanent solution to a recurring issue.

The communication encapsulated in emotions is there to help us utilize their energy in a consciously controlled fashion. Practice in heeding the message behind emotional energy will eventually allow us to manage our actions and interactions more easily—through freedom of choice, not through fearful habitual *re*-actions.

Blending science with metaphysics

Scientific research has shown that *primary emotions* appear to have a subjective component (inner recognition); a physiological component (effects on the nervous system and endocrine system, producing sweating, gooseflesh, etc.); and a behavioral component (smiling, crying, running away, etc.).

Research originally based on facial expressions, identifies six to eight primary emotions. The eight primary emotions put forward by Professor Robert Plutchik (1927–2006) in his *Wheel of Emotions* model form the foundation of the following catalog.

The catalog contains a mixture of terms we use to describe either a feeling, an emotion, or both. The framework of its construction comes from blending psychological research with metaphysical insight. It is an attempt to clarify what we are

[29]

experiencing, and what we might be doing to ourselves psychologically and physically when we experience the feeling and/or emotion.

Plutchik's primary emotions are highlighted with an asterisk. Terms beginning with a capital letter within an explanation signifies that they are included in the list.

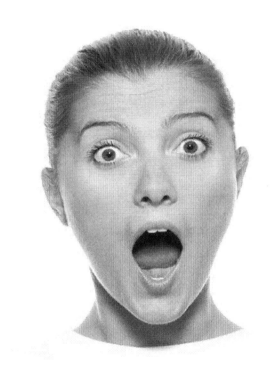

[31]

Feelings Explained: Emotions Tamed

❖ **Acceptance:** A feeling that connects us to the natural power of Divine Love (see *Glossary of Terms*). It is the basis for combating a judgmental attitude.

❖ **Aggression:** A feeling thought to be a combination of the primary emotions of Anger* and Anticipation*. Aggression is a signal generated by our body-consciousness, a surge of energy. Feelings of aggression stem from natural impulses to do with the expression of intent through creative actions. Nature displays "natural aggression" through acts such as a flower bursting from its bud, a butterfly emerging from its cocoon, and any birth process where new life comes into the physical realm.

Seth advises that we should handle feelings of aggression very quickly by turning their energy into beneficial actions, such as physical activity for the body. The problem with aggression lies with not acting quickly, thus allowing the energies to build before we release them uncontrollably through malevolent actions.

❖ **Anger*:** A scientifically recognized expression of an emotion. It begins with an emotional-signal that can rapidly introduce the emotional energy. The principle message conveyed with the emotion is that we are confining our choice of action. A belief or set of beliefs we hold with considerable electrical (emotional) charge is confining our

[32]

ability to choose how to act. We are placing blinders on our conscious-mind.

Anger is an extreme of the emotional-signal of Frustration, which arises as we mentally begin to shut down our freedom of choice. When we restrict our options to seemingly only one course of action the emotional-signal of Rage appears.

Extreme anger automatically focuses all our conscious-mind's attention on solely the outer five-senses information for working out how to act. Invariably, the outer senses do not contain enough information for the conscious-mind to come to a sound decision.

As the sensible solution on how to act comes from information that is within us, our ego-self perceives itself to be a *victim of the circumstances.* Being a victim relinquishes all responsibility for its, and thereby our, creations. If we create a release of the energies of anger through violence, we may experience subsequent emotional-signals *(such as "artificial guilt," see Guilt)* that appear to absolve us (our ego-selves) from our actions. Of course, allowing such emotional-signals to persist does nothing of the kind. It will, however, likely mask the direct *feeling* of *natural guilt,* which follows a violation. The preceding emotional-signal of Anger is not the same as the feeling of Irritation.

❖ **Anticipation***: Anticipation is a scientifically recognized expression of an emotion. It is an emotion preceded by the positive emotional-signal of Excitement, or a negative emotional-signal of nervousness—the precursor to Anxiety.

[33]

Excitement is a positive, empowering energy that helps drive the creation process in accordance with our intent and purpose. Anxiety's energy also steers our creations, but with a contrasting outcome in Expectation.

With this information in mind, it is not surprising that Abraham (Esther Hicks) suggests we foster the positive emotional-signal of Excitement in combination with the emotion of anticipation.

❖ **Anxiety:** Anxiety is an emotional-signal that announces doubt. Anxiety can escalate in intensity bringing in the emotion of Fear*.

Fearful anxiety's communication is that we are presently unable to see the choices we have available to us in working out our next actions.

We physically express anxiety in accordance with the degree of emotional energy involved. Crying and shaking, for example, are the physical expressions that signify a release of energy by our body-consciousness. Our body-consciousness does this because we are holding energy tightly within us, binding it to us and creating a physical tension. Our body-consciousness is saying, "You need to relax!"

Anxiety indicates that we are creating a *fog* of Fear in our conscious-mind that makes it increasingly difficult for us to see the choices we have available to us.

While Anger *confines* our view of the choices available, anxiety produces an obscuring mist. *We know we have choices available; we simply cannot see them clearly enough to decide.* Elias has this to add about anxiety:

[34]

"If you are experiencing anxiety, allow yourself to identify and define within yourself what is creating this expression of anxiety. As you look within yourself, what is the anxiety in relation to? Where is your attention moving? In what direction is it moving — anticipation and expectation of what you may or may not generate in the future? What are you generating within the now? For the energy that is generated in the now is what shapes the future."

❖ **Appreciation**: Appreciation is a feeling that is an expression of the natural power of Divine Love. It is the basis for instilling a Love for our Self—not simply the ego-self. As Jean Houston says, "What you appreciate, appreciates."

❖ **Compassion**: A feeling derived from the natural power of Divine Love and the exercising of our empathic set of inner senses (see *Glossary of Terms*).

❖ **Contentment:** Contentment is a *state of being* (see *Glossary of Terms*) that generates feelings such as Happiness.

❖ **Depression**: Depression begins as an emotional-signal that heralds the discounting of our creative abilities. It can escalate to an intensity of emotion that comes with the communication that we perceive ourselves to be completely powerless to create and are thus a *victim* of circumstances. Seth remarks:

> One of the strongest general causes of depression, for example, is the belief that your conscious

[35]

mind is powerless either in the face of exterior circumstances thrust upon you from without, or before strong emotional events that seem to be overwhelming from within.
(Roberts, J. (1974) *The Nature of Personal Reality: A Seth Book.* Englewood Cliffs, NJ: Prentice-Hall Inc. p. 230.)

❖ **Desire:** Desire is a feeling that emanates from our inner self in accordance with the needs of our overall Self and its determination to fully express our Self in harmony with our intent and purpose.

❖ **Disgust*:** This is a scientifically recognized expression of an emotion. The *feeling* of disgust informs our conscious-mind that the perceived action, object, or event is in sharp contrast to our beliefs and values. If the feeling persists, it turns into an emotional-signal, and may then gain further energy, reaching the status of an emotion.

The emotional message of disgust suggests that we look to our beliefs as to which of them may be in contradiction with the values highlighted by the action, object, or event.

❖ **Disappointment:** Disappointment is an emotional-signal that resembles a combination of the emotions of Surprise* and Sadness*.

Elias suggests that disappointment is an energy that quickly gathers into an emotion if we do not notice the initial signal. The signal informs our conscious-mind that a perceived event is not in line with our desires. If our

[36]

thoughts dwell on this, thus building energy, disappointment becomes an emotion with a message. The message infers that we are discounting our ability to create that which we Desire.

Disappointment arises as an automatic response to an Expectation (*see below*) that has taken an Anxiety plus Anticipation* path to manifestation. Our concentration of thought has been upon the lack of that which we Desire or upon the possible negative outcomes. Our ignorance of how we build our expectations and how they become manifest in the physical realm results in many disappointments.

❖ **Doubt:** The feeling of doubt signals a lack of Trust* in our physical self. This may stem from beliefs about our abilities or our Worthiness. The feeling of doubt precedes emotions that can quickly escalate in intensity and produce extremely debilitating conditions such as Depression. See also, Fear* and Trust*.

❖ **Envy:** Feeling envious is to do with doubting your ability to create the physical object, experience, or situation you desire that you see accomplished by another person. Instead of being appreciative of another's physical creation of say, a beautiful home, and allowing our viewing of it to reinvigorate our own creational desires, the feeling can give rise to Doubt (see above). Not to be confused with Jealousy.

To remedy envy, appreciate the emotional-signal and regard it as a reminder of what you

desire for yourself, which you will create within your own *"natural time*."*

❖ **Excitement**: As Bashar states, the *feeling* of excitement is a *direct sensing* indicating to us that what we are focusing our attention upon agrees with our spiritual path of intent and purpose. **We should therefore Trust* in this feeling.** It is a feeling that draws to us experiences that are also in line with our intent and purpose. Excitement in combination with the emotion of Anticipation* provides the momentum to project our desires into physicality.

You should not be afraid to follow your excitement. If it shifts from one thing you're doing to another, go where the strongest feeling of excitement takes you. It will lead you to the places, the people, and the situations that are in harmony with your desires.

❖ **Expectation**: An expectation is a feeling that describes a potent combination of emotional energies. We cannot classify expectation as an independent emotion as it is often an amalgamation of energies constructed from various emotions.

Here are some example combinations we easily recognize:

- Excitement plus Anticipation* produces a positive expectation of an event being in line with our intent.

- Anxiety plus Anticipation* produces Worry— expectation of a negative outcome.

[38]

- As the combination of the energies of Anticipation* and Anger* (see Aggression above) would suggest, this driving energetic potency of expectation requires direction.

  Turning our expectations into preferred outcomes is all about learning how to consciously manipulate and direct our emotional energies. We manifest our desires (and other psychic constructions) through the force of expectation.

  A concentration on thoughts alone will not bring about an expectation's materialization—at least, not until we were to spend some considerable time sustaining a purity of thought. If we wish for a Desire to become real, we need to be fully conversant with the nature of our beliefs, for it is our beliefs that affect an expectation's likelihood of coming to fruition.

- ❖ **Fear***: Fear is a scientifically recognized expression of an emotion. Like Love, fear expresses itself through all forms of information transfer. It can come as a direct *Impulse* to act (fight or flight) or express itself through an emotional-signal that leads to an emotion. This spectrum of expression indicates that fear is more to do with our current state of being and is a primary means to get us to act immediately.

  Fear as an Impulse (a direct sensing and information transfer), happens in conjunction with our will to survive; as an emotional-signal, it alerts us to self-doubt arising within us (see Anxiety); and the full-blown emotion of fear produces all manner of debilitating symptoms across the physiological and psychological systems of our Self.

[39]

It is important to note that fear is not part of our psychological structuring, it is generated *by* our psychological structuring—namely the beliefs we hold, and the thoughts we nurture.

Fears can arise from our misinterpretation of what *is* a basic psychological structure guiding our actions – the survival of Consciousness. *Our* consciousness translates this quality of Consciousness into basic physical terms—forming a psychological structure that ensures our survival within the physical plane of existence. When energy associated with this primordial drive channels through us as an *impulse*, we act immediately, *un*-consciously, and without thinking. Thank goodness!

However, when "fearful" energy traverses through us as an emotional-signal followed by an emotion, we are, in the moment, consciously accessing a distortionary element in our psychological structure that mistranslates this fundamental drive for survival. Our inability to correctly decipher the nuances of inner data involved with this drive often generates fear—and Hatred.

The overall problem of fear has much to do with the ego-self's refusal to incorporate subconscious information and experiences supplied by the inner self. Thus, it is the ego-self's *lack of understanding that generates fear,* which then diminishes our connection to the natural power of Divine Love. Fear tells of our disconnection from Divine Love (*see Love*)—which makes it imperative that we resolve and *understand* what beliefs are generating the fear.

The experience of fearfulness comes with the basic message that we are generating a *lack of Trust** within ourselves.

❖ **Forgiveness**: This feeling originates as an *Impulse* (direct communication from our Essence self) to act in a *compassionate* way. Feelings of hurt generate the impulse of forgiveness—we, or most likely someone else, has literally hurt our feelings (our psychological structuring) or our physical creations (our body, or another physical construct of our own creation).

The impulse directs us to act compassionately, *in the first instance*, toward Self. This is because it relates to our own creative abilities and **the natural principle of Creation (see *Glossary of Terms* for more about the *Natural Principles*)**.

The original impulse to act is an attempt to remind us that we create *all* of our reality, even the hurtful, negative events. If we perceive another party to be the perpetrator of any hurt to us, realize that they have co-opted with us in *our* creation. They are reflecting a need for us to examine our feelings and beliefs that associate with the hurtful event and attend to them.

To *blame* others for *any* experience that is not to our liking, puts our creative power outside of ourselves, denigrates the other party's co-creative abilities, and proclaims us a *victim*. As with Anger, being a victim relinquishes all responsibility for our creations. Blaming yourself thus denigrates our own creative abilities and is an

[41]

admission that we do not belief we can create the reality we prefer.

Forgiveness is not about *correcting* a hurt in the manner we are used to—forgive and forget. When we understand the impulse for what it is, directing us to be compassionate, then be so—in our forgiveness of our self and others.

Forgiveness will also exercise our power of Appreciation. We should learn to appreciate a seemingly "negative" co-creation for what it brings to us. **Compassion and Appreciation then combine in a genuine expression of forgiveness.**

Appreciate that the other party helped bring this feeling to us for the purposes of our own learning—the craft of conscious creating—and growth.

❖ **Freedom:** A feeling of freedom indicates a psychological state that is allowing source energy to flow freely through our Self in its natural manner. That natural manner is in accordance with our intent and purpose.

❖ **Frustration:** Frustration begins as an emotional-signal that brings our attention to an element within our awareness that we perceive to be reflecting some form of lack in our physical self and our creative abilities.

This signal of lack can relate to many different ways of discounting our self: that we lack the ability to choose or make a decision, are not good enough, not wealthy enough, not strong enough, not quick enough, not *enough* in some way.

If the signal grows, through thought, into the emotion of frustration, it can result in a considerable belittling of our self.

The communication with any emotional energy attracted by our thinking indicates that our conscious-mind is confused as to the nature of its choices for action; which, as energy builds, can attract both the emotional-signal of Anxiety, and the emotion of Anger*.

We often view frustration as a "normal" state because we experience it so often.

Anger* is the extreme of frustration, an emotion that indicates the perceived confusion over choices is turning into a perception of no choice at all.

❖ **Grief:** See **Sadness*/Sorrow**.

❖ **Guilt**: It is important to remember that guilt takes two forms – *artificial guilt* and *natural guilt*.

Artificial guilt stems from the transgression of laws and ethical codes constructed as part of a particular belief system. For example, feeling guilty about a sexual act (that is consensual and enjoyed by the parties involved) you've performed because you *believe* it to be "sinful" (outside the union of marriage) produces artificial guilt.

Natural guilt is an instinctive psychological mechanism to protect against our physical self continually committing acts of violation.

The *feeling* is a direct sensing from our inner self to our conscious-mind that we are about to, are in the process

[43]

of, or have just, violated the natural principles underpinning the vitality of Divine Love.

The *emotion* of natural guilt is the result of transgressing the vitality of Divine Love. It provides us with the energy to make amends if possible and the message to closely exam our beliefs regarding the act in question. Natural guilt will occur if our actions violate our physical self or another physical expression of Consciousness.

Rape, for example, is a violating action producing natural guilt. If the perpetrator of this action does not experience the feeling or the emotion of natural guilt (which invokes feelings of Remorse – *see below*), or they repress the emotion's energy, a psychotic disorder either exists or can develop.

❖ **Happiness**: The feeling of happiness is entirely reliant upon our interpretation of an experience. We generate happiness when we create an experience that is in accordance with our Desire and intent. The intensity of happiness is proportional to the degree to which the experience reflects the detail of our Desire and synchronizes with our intent and purpose.

The *continuity* (our translation of *"durability,"* one of Seth's "inner laws of the universe") of our happiness rests upon how often we can remain in harmony with our overall intent and purpose.

For example, imagining that great financial abundance will make us happy, and on its appearance, it does so only fleetingly, indicates that our imagination generated a *Want* for financial abundance rather than a sincere Desire for

[44]

what financial abundance would bring us—ultimately, the ability to do what we wish to do, when we wish to do it.

To many of us happiness is an illusory experience. Elias remarks that this is because we know happiness to be pleasurable, and we have many beliefs that block the experience simply because of this knowledge.

Any pleasurable feeling, such as happiness, comes directly from our Essence self to tell us that we are currently experiencing Self-Fulfillment.

Disappointment (*see above*) is a feeling closely related to happiness as it gives indication of when an experience is not in line with our Desire.

❖ **Hatred**: Hatred begins as a feeling before exploiting an emotion for its energy. It is the result of a psychological manipulation of the emotion of Fear*.

As with Fear*, hatred is to do with our misinterpretation of the quality or drive within Consciousness to maintain existence (we translate this as "survive"). Misconceptions plague our attempts to translate this quality of Consciousness into a cohesive psychological structure within our own psyche.

Depending on the degree of distortion or errors in our own psychological construction, this structure then affects, detrimentally, our physical creations. Errors in translation may become habitual and the distortions can influence other psychological structures. We integrate the errors into our perception.

[45]

Hate is not so much the opposite of love, as the separation of the physical self from the natural power of Divine Love and the inner senses that operate within it.

Hate as an emotion highlights our seeming separation from Consciousness. Our ego-self's perception of separation generates a Fear* of losing its personal identity, of returning to the fold (on physical death), of being One again with Consciousness. Beware the natural inner *law of attraction* when it comes to hate—for if we hate, we will attract hate.

❖ **Hope**: The feeling of hope associates with optimism, a combination of the emotions of Anticipation* and Joy*.

A review of Anticipation* shows that this emotion can involve either Anxiety or Excitement in the steering of its energies. Hope can therefore take two contrasting routes.

The first route is when the emphasis of our thoughts, feelings, and emotions center on the lack of our desired manifestation or the negativity of the current situation. It is then that our Anticipation* involves the confounding energies of Anxiety in any Expectation.

The other route involves maintaining a focus on the desired positive change in the situation. Focusing on the Desire invokes feelings of Excitement in our Anticipation*. Such grounding feelings and emotions marry readily with Joy* to produce an Expectation far more capable of creating the outcome we "hope" for.

❖ **Impatience:** Impatience is a feeling that signals to our conscious-mind that we are not allowing the energies that

[46]

coalesce to form our desired reality to flow freely within *natural time.*

This feeling relates to the emotion of Trust*--of our Self and our creative abilities. Impatience is a symptom of our ego-self's attempt to force a desired probable event outside of its natural timing.

❖ **Impulse**: Neither a feeling nor an emotion, an impulse is a direct energy communication, an *instructional* prompting, from our Essence self that gets our physical self to act before the intervention of complicating thoughts or feelings.

Impulses are lifelong communications directing our actions. They constitute a form of language used by our inner self, our physical self's guardian, to act with immediacy.

We mistrust impulses because of established core beliefs that misinterpret the nature of the subconscious and misunderstand our natural drive for survival.

Even though our belief systems tell us to mistrust them, *impulses are not harmful to us.* Instead of ignoring or repressing impulses, trust that following them without too much analysis by the conscious-mind will be of benefit.

Committing a violation has nothing to do with *natural* impulses. Acts of violation of a natural principle or a societal law are often blamed on "an impulse," when in fact they are instigated by mischievous, malevolent, or pathological patterns of thought.

❖ **Irritation**: A feeling often confused with Anger*, irritation can accrue an energy potential as elevated as the emotion of

[47]

Anger, however, it is a quite different energy configuration. The difference is that irritation empowers us, whereas Anger disempowers us.

Even though they feel very much alike, one way of separating them is to notice whether we have paused in our actions to consider our options. This would be a sign that we are *irritated* rather than angry.

Irritation usually stops us in our tracks and makes us consider the situation and our choices for action. Anger is the emotion that has us believe, without consideration, that there are few choices, if any, available.

We *always* have choices in any situation, considering them is empowering as we are consciously in charge of our choices and subsequent actions. Anger disempowers us as it narrows or takes away completely conscious choice, replacing it with a reaction.

Anger, at best, pushes us into a choice that is not genuinely in line with our desires or intent; irritation engages our imagination. Irritation sees to it that the circumstances do not dictate how we should act and that we maintain a choice on how to proceed.

❖ **Jealousy**: Whereas Envy is to do with desire for another's physical manifestations, jealousy is to with desiring another's manifested relationship. We are, if you will, envious of the relationship someone has with another. As with Envy, jealousy is a feeling that is disparaging our creational ability to form or attract loving and intimate relationships.

[48]

The emotion of Trust* (in yourself) is at the core of jealousy. Jealousy is a feeling that can easily gain energy and become emotionally charged.

❖ **Joy***: Joy is a scientifically recognized primary emotion. It begins as a feeling that can escalate its intensity to emotion status. The feeling signals that in this moment we are validating and appreciating our self.

The emotion communicates that we are exercising a Trust* in our self, an acknowledgement that we are expressing ourselves freely in our choices and in accordance with the natural principles encapsulated by the power of Divine Love.

Abraham states that while the basis of life is freedom, joy is the true *objective* of life.

Joy is the feeling and emotion that informs us that we are freely expressing our personality in alignment with our intent and purpose.

❖ **Love**: Science suggests that love is a feeling that is a combination of the emotions of Joy* and Trust*.

From the metaphysical standpoint, love is neither a feeling nor an emotion, it is more a *state of being*. We can attain this state of being when our *vibrational signature* *(see Feeling-Tone in Glossary of Terms)* is in harmony with the frequencies that define the vital force of Consciousness— Divine Love.

Human love is our attempt to interpret the qualities of Divine Love.

[49]

Divine Love is an expansive state that encompasses, and can be expressed by, many feelings and emotions. Omni's description, *"In essence, it is a total knowing, Acceptance, and Appreciation of what is,"* appears to be the most reasonable and succinct interpretation of the qualities of Divine Love.

❖ **Pain**: Pain is of great interest to science as it assumes that the brain somehow generates the physical symptom. Metaphysical literature informs us that pain, whether physical, emotional, or psychological, is a nonphysical based *feeling* which our inner self and/or body-consciousness generates.

Physical pain is a direct communication to our conscious-mind from our inner self, in cooperation with the body-consciousness, that immediate action is required.

An enduring physical pain, along with emotional and psychological pain, communicates that our beliefs need review and adjustment.

Pain, as with any feeling, passes through our *perception*. It is our perception that identifies whether the feeling is positive or negative in nature; which is why we can experience a physical pain as both positive (pleasurable) and negative (unpleasant).

❖ **Rage**: Rage is an emotional-signal that arises out of the highly charged emotion of Anger*. When our choice of action appears to have narrowed to only one or two options the feeling of rage alerts us to this so that we might break our pattern of thought before we act recklessly.

❖ **Remorse**: A feeling thought to be a combination of Sadness* and Disgust*. It is a feeling that stems from natural guilt, thereby invoking the emotions of Sadness* and Disgust* at one's actions.

These combined emotions communicate that it is essential that we take time to look within and deal with beliefs that have become so inappropriate as to be pathological or life threatening.

❖ **Sadness*/Sorrow**: Science recognizes sadness as a primary emotion. Sadness is the *emotional-signal*, which may, or may not lead to the emotion of *sorrow*.

Sadness usually signals the loss of a preferred creation from our perception of reality. This could be a cherished object, an abandoned idea or concept, a beloved animal or plant, or of course, a fellow human being.

When the loss appears to have obvious permanence, as in physical death, the signal of sadness may evoke the emotion of sorrow. We can think of sorrow as the emotion that steps in to prolong the feeling of sadness.

Our mental blurring of the differing energies of the signal of sadness with the emotion of sorrow leads to a confused understanding of their information content.

The signal of sadness also implies that we perceive a limitation of our choices. When we are just dealing with the emotional-signal, there is recognition of loss, but the underlying communication is suggesting that if we employ

[51]

the emotion of sorrow, we may enter into some type of denial of our self and our creative abilities. This may relate to actions we've taken, to our future choice of actions, or to our *freedom* to act.

Remember that anger and anxiety are emotional states which also carry the message that we are subconsciously perceiving a limitation of choice. Sadness contains this subconscious information, but when sorrow comes into the reckoning, a greater subtlety of meaning emerges—largely missed by most of us.

When sorrow enters the picture, part of the message comes from our Essence self. *It* is *feeling sad* for our physical self! Our Essence is sad that we are not using the sorrowful experience to learn more about our *co-creative abilities*. In the case of the death of a loved one, it is sad that we do not understand that physical death is not the end to that person or creature's existence, or their influence upon our creations.

Sadness is the signal that the loved one was of value to us in the co-creation of our reality. It is a signal designed to bring our mind into a state of *appreciation* (an expression of Divine Love) of the value of the other's contribution to our life. Sadness is thereby the feeling that has us recognize and appreciate that in *cooperation* (a natural principle) with this other person or creature we were able to co-create mutually beneficial experiences.

The fact that the other no longer chooses to *directly* participate in our physical reality, appears to our ego-self to put a limit on our further choices in life, when actually the event signals an opening of choices, more self-

[52]

empowerment, and more clarity in relation to our Self. (*Imagine that the person leaving the physical domain is saying, "I trust that you don't need my help anymore in the creation of your reality. You'll do fine without me or with someone new."*)

Grieving is a natural process that releases the ego-self's feeling of sadness along with dissipating the emotional energy that follows as the ego-self comes to terms with the ending of the co-created physical experience. Crying is a physical symptom of that energy release.

❖ **Stress:** Stress occurs when we fail to recognize emotional-signals sent from our inner self, which inform us of the lack of *naturalness* in our actions. Emotional-signals, unrecognized, are apt to build in number and intensity in our subconscious. Failure to acknowledge their existence, and address the emotional energies that associate with them, creates a highly debilitating effect upon our psychological and physiological systems.

Extreme stress, that is, storing emotional-signals and other feelings over time, can eventually result in a nervous breakdown.

❖ **Surprise*:** Surprise is a scientifically recognized primary emotion—the opposite of Anticipation*. Metaphysical sources tell us that surprise is a *feeling*, which sweeps over us to inform us that the created event was not within our normal parameters of Expectation. We can think of it as a reminder to us that our expectations do not have to constrain our creative abilities.

[53]

❖ **Trust***: This is a scientifically recognized emotion. Trust though, according to channeled information, is not actually an emotion, it is a state of being resulting from an affinity with Divine Love. *(Remember that Fear* tells of our disconnection from Divine Love.)* Attuning to Divine Love incorporates *feelings* of trust within us for our Self and our perception of reality.

Expressing trust is an expression of our personal Freedom (the basis of life) to allow the natural flow of energy to move unencumbered along our chosen path of intent. In doing so, we are trusting that the probabilities relating to our Desire have been set in motion and their manifestation does not necessarily require any further injection of energy, such as that provided by an emotion. We trust in the natural flow of universal energy to manifest our Desire in *natural time.*

The Elias messages often focus on trusting our Self because, "You shall not betray yourself!"

Yes, it is particularly difficult to trust our Self when we are under constant pressure from others to trust in them. Making things more difficult still is an ego-self that trusts only the information brought to it by our physical senses, and the knowledge it has contorted to fit within its belief systems.

Know that when others proclaim that you should trust in the universe, this will indeed help you to some degree as it *is* the universe—Consciousness—that provides the ultimate state of Trust through Divine Love.

[54]

As we are a "portion" of Consciousness, trust is therefore implicit to the nature of our Self.

❖ **Vulnerable**: The feeling of vulnerability signals our conscious-mind that we are *open to receive* energy and information. We label this feeling as "negative" as we associate being open to receive as being open to violation, or without adequate protection. We assign this *belief* to the feeling, thus generating the energy potential of the emotion of Fear*.

This habitual action conceals the feeling's good intent to inform us that in the present moment we are receptive to any form of feedback about our creations.

❖ **Want:** A want is a feeling that our ego-self generates when information gathered by the outer senses filters through our belief systems. Because of the nature of belief systems, a Desire (generated by our inner self and our inner senses) can be misinterpreted as a want and vice versa.

❖ **Worry**: This is a feeling that combines Anxiety with Anticipation* – an Expectation of a negative creation. It's worth remembering Abraham's definition of worry if we find ourselves doing it: "Worrying is using your imagination to create that which you do not want."

Of course, worrying, via anxiety, can lead to a fearful emotion. The message of the emotion is that we are perpetuating a lack of Trust* in our Self, and our ability to create that which we Desire. We are channeling our energies toward a negative outcome via a negative Expectation.

[55]

To quell worrying thoughts, focus your attention upon an excited Anticipation of a preferred outcome.

❖ **Worthiness**: To feel "unworthy" is to deny who you are. It's a feeling that can form a psychological dam holding back the natural flow of Source energy and the energies of feelings and emotions that seek expression through your physical self.

These energies strive to have you express your uniqueness, your intent, your creativity, and your purpose in life. Feeling unworthy drives your Essence self to tears!

This happens as your Essence self knows that as an individuated expression of Consciousness your right to exist requires no justification. There is no measure of worthiness or validity for *your* consciousness within Consciousness as it is a part of It. Consciousness does not create something within All That Is for no reason. Consequently, everything within All That Is is important to It. To question your worth is to question the worth of Consciousness. **Therefore, your very existence is proof enough that you have both value and worth.**

Seth has this to add:

If you believe that you are of little merit, inferior and filled with guilt, then you may react in several ways according to your personal background and the framework in which you accepted those beliefs. You may be terrified of aggressive feelings because [it seems] others so

[56]

much more powerful than you could retaliate. If you believe that all such thoughts are wrong, you will inhibit them and feel all the more guilty— which will generate aggressiveness against yourself and further deepen your sense of unworthiness.

(Roberts, J. (1974) *The Nature of Personal Reality: A Seth Book.* Englewood Cliffs, NJ: Prentice-Hall Inc. p. 231.)

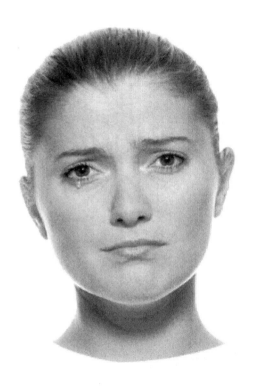

What You're Doing to Your Self

In my book *It's About You: Know Your Self*, it is made evident that for someone to pursue a healthy and purposeful life one must first, indeed, know thy Self.

Knowing your Self relates to the physical and spiritual aspects that constitute the overall "Self," with particular regard to the psychological energies such as thoughts, beliefs, feelings and emotions that not only mold our personality, but also govern and form the way we create our personal reality.

Once we're able to accept the central premise—that our beliefs are the crucial factor in the formation of our reality—we can better understand and utilize the functions of our feelings and emotions and begin repairing and reformulating those beliefs that prevent us from creating our preferred reality.

The generation of negative feelings and emotions during an experience points us in the direction of one or two ways in which we are denigrating our Self. What we are denigrating is usually to do with our *ability to create* our preferred reality.

Once we're clearer on what emotion/s we're dealing with, we can then explore the message of an emotion to help us root out the problematic belief/s that are at work.

The 3Ds – Dissing, Denial, Distrust

There are essentially three forms of self-denigration, which I've labeled the "3Ds":

1. **Dissing of Self** – meaning that we are being *disrespectful* to our Self. We are discounting and devaluing our Self—

[58]

thus *violating* our Self—which subsequently undermines our self-esteem. (Non-violation is one of the natural principles outlined in Book I of this *Being Human* series— see the *Glossary of Terms*.)

Feelings and emotions involved with dissing include:

Dis-appointment! A self-imposed promotion of self-dissing. Discounting your ability to create what you desire.

Envy. Doubting your ability to create the physical object, experience, or situation you desire that you see accomplished by another person.

Guilt. Guilt is to do with devaluing your Self. It's important to identify whether you are feeling *natural* or *artificial* guilt. Linked to the emotion of **Remorse**.

2. **Denial of Self** – meaning that we are denying our creational abilities because we don't *believe* we create our reality and are thus a *victim* of the circumstances.

Feelings and emotions involved with denial of Self:

Anxiety. The emotional-signal of anxiety announces doubt. **Doubt** can escalate into the emotion of **Fear**. Anxiety clouds your vision when trying to make a choice.

Depression. This begins with an emotional-signal that heralds the discounting of your creational abilities. Depression can elevate anxiety levels to such a degree that the Throat chakra (see *Glossary of Terms*) center becomes blocked.

Anger. Anger's message is that a belief is narrowing down our choice of action.

Sadness and Sorrow. The *feeling* of sadness signals some type of denial of our Self and our creative abilities. Sorrow, the emotion, relates to discounting our *co-creative* capabilities.

Unworthiness. Feeling a lack of self-worth is to do with denying who you are—a uniquely worthy expression of Consciousness.

3. **Distrust of Self** – which relates to believing we are separated from the vital life force of Divine Love.

Feelings and emotions associated with distrust of Self:

Fear. Survival impulse aside, fear is the primary way of telling your ego-self that you are not trusting in you being a part of Consciousness. It is the ego-self's ultimate feeling of disconnection or separation from Source.

Hatred. Feelings and emotions that relate to misconceptions about survival and our separation from Source.

Impatience. Not trusting in "natural time."

Trust. The more we trust in our Self, the more we are in alignment with Divine Love. Why? Because All That Is, which includes our Self, is an expression of Consciousness. Trusting in our Self is trusting in Consciousness to steer us along our unique, purposeful path of learning.

Vulnerable. A feeling misinterpreted because of a belief that to be vulnerable is to be open to violation. Fear stems from it, which is distrusting of Self once again.

Worry. Fixating upon fearful feelings.

It is worth noting that feelings of depression, which can engage emotional energy if not attended to, fall within all three of the ways in which we denigrate our Self. This is why it can be so debilitating—a true case of dis-ability—dis-abling one's creational abilities to such an extent that the natural principle of Creativity (see *Glossary of Terms*) is psychologically quashed within us.

What To Do About The 3Ds

How to dissipate the energies of negative feelings and emotions

By far the easiest and most self-empowering way of addressing negative feelings and emotions is a simple technique developed originally by Gary Craig called Emotional Freedom Techniques, now widely known as EFT or simply "tapping."

To get started with EFT, a lifelong tool for dissipating negative emotional energy, there is a free one sheet PDF document on the EFT basics available at this URL:

https://cwejohnson.com/wp-content/uploads/2015/12/Basic-Short-Cut-Version-of-EFT.pdf

I recommend you see a certified practitioner to clarify its use in the long term and if wanting to deal with long-standing emotional conditions. You can find practitioners and training in the use of EFT at these recommended websites:

emofree.com (Gary Craig's website.)
eftuniverse.com
thetappingsolution.com
theeftcentre.com (UK)

My own research and experience with EFT have led to the development of an EFT protocol specifically targeting issues to do with self-worth. Lack of self-worth appears to be highly prevalent within the global populous, indicating that problematic beliefs associated with worthiness are deeply entrenched within the collective psyche of humanity at present. In view of the many centuries of religious, political, and educational doctrine insidiously designed to subjugate and contain an individual's feelings of powerfulness—most notably in regard to women—it is hardly surprising to find lack of self-worth at the core of our being.

In light of this, while you familiarize yourself with the basics of using EFT on any personal emotional issues you may have, I suggest you download and practice "**A Core EFT Exercise: Tapping for Self-Worth**" a few times. You'll be pleasantly surprised at the boost to your confidence it brings. The PDF is available at the **cwejohnson.com/offerings** page.

Abraham suggests this simple exercise

As you are moving through your day, try this exercise. When you find yourself feeling negative emotion or physical sensation, which is just an exaggeration of resistance in your body, go to a piece of paper, or you can write it in your computer, but write it. And write:

Subject: And then write what you think this subject is, just a very brief description.

And then write:

Current Set Point: And then think around the subject and it won't be hard because you're already thinking around it, that's why you are having the emotion. Think around the subject and just even talk out loud or write it is even better. Write what's rolling through your mind on the subject that has produced the emotion. And as you write each statement, ask yourself as the statements come, **"What's the emotion that describes this?"** And you'll find yourself where you are on the vibrational meter, finding words that are all similar, that mean sort of the same thing. And then say, My Current Emotional Set Point is: And then write whatever it is. Then write:

My Emotional Goal, not My Physical Body Improvement Goal, write **My Emotional Goal:**

Now, of course, the optimum emotional goal would be ecstasy or passion or enthusiasm. But don't ask for an emotional goal that's very far from where you are. Ask for an emotional goal that is not so far from where you are. And then keep writing, trying to find sentences and statements and memories that give you that improved feeling. And when the feeling is improved, now write:

Current Emotional Set Point: And put the new statement there. And then, if you have time, continue the process and you will be amazed how, in this writing process, in this focus on how I feel, and focus upon what thoughts are producing the feelings setting, you are sitting in, you can move up this emotional scale fast. And every day you do it, you will feel less stiff. It is our promise to you.

(Abraham-Hicks. Orlando FL., December.20, 2003.)

[64]

Your personal call to action

According to more than one metaphysical source, the Shift has begun to accelerate recently. The decade from 2016 through 2026 will see dramatic changes for humanity in how we live our lives. There will be those "called" (by their inner selves) to help others negotiate this momentous time—you may be one such person.

If your inner self has other things planned for you, then your study and adoption of the natural principles (see *Also by Chris W.E. Johnson* at the back of this book) at least as the foundation of your mental outlook is quite sufficient to have a beneficial effect upon the entire Shift process. You can proudly say to your grandchildren that you did your bit in the Shift— you shifted your own mind-set and added to the psychological critical mass required to bring about humanity's collective new worldview.

If you want to take things further, learn more and be proactive—register your email address at my website **cwejohnson.com** to receive my newsletters. If you want to find out more about other people involved with exploring what the Shift means to humanity, visit this page on my website:

cwejohnson.com/about/keep-up-with-our-shift-in-consciousness/

Fear and the Shift

Events associated with the Shift will inevitably generate fears within us. This is because our personal belief systems need to change in like manner to what's happening in our collective psyche.

The content of this book will aid you in reformulating your beliefs so that you experience less fear as we traverse the Shift.

We can begin to conquer our fears by adopting a mind-set that has, at its foundational core, the natural principles. We're not having to construct a whole new foundation. The principles have been there all along; it's just that our ego-selves have been off experimenting with less altruistic mind-sets, not knowing that such experimentation disconnects us from Source.

Practice the Principles. It may take some time before you don't have to catch your ego-self reverting back to its selfish, judgmental, complaining norm. Have fun with it though. Keep in mind that it's your ego-self that's frightened, not the *real* you!

Notice how you are *feeling* **in any situation.** Is there a smidgeon of fear mixed in? Remind yourself that fear is behind any negative feeling—anger, anxiety, aggression, doubt, frustration, guilt, impatience, etc. See if you can **recognize and identify the beliefs** you have that appear to be initiating the negative feeling.

You then need to address those beliefs. That is, begin to dissipate the emotional charge that reinforces their importance to you. **You can do this using the basic EFT procedure** *(see the URL mentioned above).* Once you have made a start with addressing your belief systems, you'll find that you'll quickly begin to accept, allow, and appreciate yourself more— including your misguided, but doing the best it can with a flaky belief system, ego-self.

Here are some shifty symptoms. If any resonate with you,

[66]

download and follow the directions on the basic EFT procedure when addressing these issues:

❖ **Feeling overwhelmed** a lot of the time.

❖ **A feeling of generalized anxiety**, overly anxious of what *might happen* to you or your loved ones.

❖ **Losing patience more often**—with yourself and others.

❖ **A feeling of loneliness or disconnectedness** from others—despite having plenty of friends and family.

In conclusion

In the coming years, we move from ego-self-awareness to whole Self-awareness. We progress from the ego's reflections on its little-self, prone to misconceptions, fears, and habitual reactions, to a *Whole Self-reflective* ability. Our Self-reflective focus will be upon reading the communication of emotions and acting upon these instead of focusing on only the emotional-signals that precede them. We will come to realize that emotions are the life force of this physical plane, as they are integral to its expression *through* our Selves.

We need to train our ego-selves to allow emotions to flow through us with acceptance. They are, after all, *energy in motion* (E-motion), they will pass, and others will replace them.

A concluding message from our channeled friend Omni:

Many of you have for so long held to the belief that the path to God or to enlightenment is the path of suffering. Suffering has served in teaching you all about who you are not and what you do not want.

The new teacher is joy. It is not that joy is new, but that you are only now awakening to it, for your evolution has taken you to the stage where you can feel the true essence of your soul. This is truly a new dawn, this is the return of the Christ, this is the awakening of the God/Goddess within, this is the dawning of a new age.

(Omni (John L. Payne) (2001) *Omni Reveals the Four Principles of Creation*. Forres, Scotland: Findhorn Press. p. 96.)

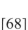

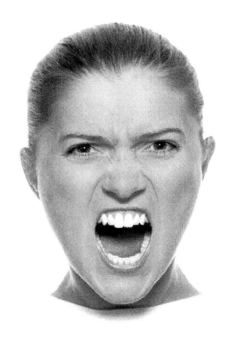

[69]

References and Resources

References

Abraham – Esther Hicks channels Abraham. For more on Abraham go to **abraham-hicks.com.**

Bashar – Darryl Anka channels Bashar. For more on Bashar go to **bashar.org.**

Elias – Mary Ennis channels Elias. For more on Elias go to **eliasweb.org or eliasforum.org.**

Omni – John L. Payne channels Omni. For more on Omni and John go to **familyconstellations.net.**

Seth – Jane Roberts channeled Seth until her death in 1984. For more information on the Seth material, and a comparative overview with the Elias transcripts, go to **newworldview.com/freebies/sethmaterial.**

Resources

Visit my website (**cwejohnson.com**) for more information and to follow up on what you've learned from this book. Register your name and email address to keep informed of news and events. As a thank you for registering, you will receive a handy PDF sheet that summarizes the **10 Natural Principles.**

Go to the **Offerings page** to freely download:

❖ **A PDF sheet of the basic EFT** (Emotional Freedom Techniques) procedure.

❖ **A Core EFT Exercise.** The script for using EFT to deal

with issues relating to lack of self-worth. You will need to register as a Subscriber to access this document. If you don't want to do that, email me at **info@cwejohnson.com** and ask me to send you a copy.

❖ **Lots of other downloads** pertaining to my book *It's About You! Know Your Self: A New Edition.* There's a link to purchase.

❖ There's also a link to purchase *How to be in Divine Love: 10½ Principles That Will Make You a Happy Purposeful Person* on the Offerings page.

Glossary of Terms

A term in **bold emphasis** within an explanation indicates that the term is included in this glossary.

Base chakra – This chakra center processes information pertaining to our spiritual self. Information received relates to our physical self's relationship to nature, to our **Essence self**, and to **Consciousness** itself. **Empathic inner senses** are integral to the relay of this information.

Belief systems – The various and many beliefs organized by individuals and groups into core topics that dominate our thinking. These systems are organic in nature, constantly overlapping and interacting with each other.

Body-consciousness – Our body-consciousness is an electromagnetic "layer" to our physical self that works within the **subconscious area** of our **mind**. It maintains all the processing systems of our physical self.

Conscious-mind – The hyphenated term used by the author to differentiate the chosen mind made conscious by the **ego-self** from the **collection of minds** within the **subconscious**.

Consciousness/consciousness – Consciousness with a capital C is the author's preferred term for the intelligent force that patterns energy into perceivable expressions. It is an alternative term for All That Is, God, Source, or any such term that refers to a "higher," absolute, omnipresent influence upon the Cosmos. Consciousness with a small c, as in human *consciousness* or your *consciousness,* means to convey an individuated expression of capital-C Consciousness.

Core beliefs – A core belief is one that we deem to be true or an unquestionable fact. Elias refers to a set of ten fundamental **belief** *systems* that are at the core of our thinking. We can think of them as *subject themes* that cover the entirety of our thought processing.

Creativity – one of the **natural principles** described in *How to be in Divine Love: 10½ Principles That Will Make You a Happy Purposeful Person.* Book I in the *"Being Human"* series.

Divine Love – The term given to the all-pervasive force that describes the vitality of **Consciousness.** "Value Fulfillment" is the term most often used by Seth.

Ego-self – The ego or ego-self is a psychological structure within the physical self for interpreting what we perceive in the physical field.

Electric field – The electric field is a term used to encompass a variety of electromagnetic energy fields based in the dimension of existence "closest" to the physical dimension.

Emotion/s – The independent energy form that, as a bare minimum, provides our physical self with additional energy for action and information on our inner state of being. It invariably includes with its dispatch essential

[73]

information on our current psychological structuring—
usually relating to our beliefs.

Emotional-signal – The special type of feeling that signals the
imminent onset of an **emotion**.

Empathic inner senses – The empathic inner senses allow you
to intuitively know the *being-ness* of any structure within
your field of perception. Employing these **inner senses** in
the perception of another organic structure, such as a tree,
an animal, or another person, stimulates a far greater
appreciation and compassion for that expression of
Consciousness.

Essence/Essence self – terms used by the author to refer to the
nonphysical or spiritual self.

Feeling/s – A signal that precedes direct transfer of information
and/or energy to the **conscious-mind** and physiological
systems.

Feeling-tone/Tonal frequency – Expressions used to describe
the combined frequencies of the thoughts, beliefs, feelings,
and emotional energies maintained by our **personality**.
This combination of frequencies, when also combined
with the primal tone of our **Essence self** constitutes our
vibrational signature.

Garden of Beliefs – The Garden of Beliefs is a metaphor
introduced by the author to describe the **subconscious**
"place" within the **mind** where thoughts, beliefs, and
emotions combine to produce our *emotional climate*. Our
emotional climate describes the overall state of our

[74]

personality's mood.

Impressions – Impressions are a subtle form of communication relayed to the **conscious-mind** from our **inner self**. Often dismissed too readily as unreliable figments of the imagination or wishful thinking, they appear as random thoughts but are motivated from within to present you with rudimentary information about an object in question.

Impulses – Impulses are direct instructional prompts to the **conscious-mind**, emanating from our **Essence self**, for us to act in a certain way. Their function is to bypass the thought processing mechanism which may prevent us from acting.

Inner self – Our inner self acts as an emissary to our **Essence**. It is that part of our **Essence self** that focuses upon looking after and assisting our physical self as it explores and experiences the physical world.

Inner senses – A set of senses that our **inner self** utilizes in providing our **ego-self**'s **conscious-mind** with information from the spiritual domain.

Intent and purpose – Intent is a directional force within and part of **Consciousness**. It is the impetus by which it explores itself. This translates to human consciousness as directional paths of learning for exploring *our* Self. Purpose refers to the unique goal of learning that our **Essence** plans for us to attain in our lifetime.

Mind/collection of minds – Our mind is the portion of the psyche, situated within our **Essence**, most actively involved with our **inner self** in maintaining our physical existence. According to Seth, we have a collection of minds available to us that can be made the **conscious-mind**, in accordance with the circumstances.

Natural guilt – Natural guilt results from transgressing the primary natural principle of non-violation. The feeling of natural guilt is essentially a direct message from our inner self signaling our conscious-mind that such a transgression has occurred. Heed the message by ceasing whatever has initiated this feeling. This is primarily for *our* benefit, as well as any other party involved.

Natural principles – a set of principles by which **Consciousness** operates when expressing itself through the medium of human consciousness in physicality. The natural principles describe the creation process of **Divine Love** as interpreted through human consciousness. Book I of the *"Being Human"* series, *How to be in Divine Love: 10½ Principles That Will Make You a Happy, Purposeful Person,* explores and explains these principles for conscious living.

Natural time - Natural time refers to natural rhythms and cycles involved in the expression of **Consciousness** in the physical realm. Seasonal cycles and physiological cycles are examples of actions that obey natural time.

Non-violation – A violation is a deliberate act to end, harm, or undermine the physical or psychological freedom of another expression of **Consciousness**.

Remember it is possible to violate not just another person

or living thing, but an object, a space, or an environment. If unsure of where your actions stand, ask yourself, "Am I being respectful?"

Refer to: *How to be in Divine Love: 10½ Principles That Will Make You a Happy, Purposeful Person.*

Personality – Our personality is an electrically encoded counterpart to our **ego-self**. From a linear-time perspective it "begins" life along with our ego-self. It has a constantly (both in physical time and outside of it) changing and evolving nature. Its "form" is electrical in quality, residing within the electrical dimension of action. Our personality maintains a unique **tonal frequency**.

Personal intent – Personal intent is the potential we hold to fulfill our own spiritual ambitions within the pool of probabilities chosen by our **Essence self** for our current lifetime.

Shift in consciousness/Shift – A term much used in the Body/Mind/Spirit movement that relates to the evolutionary changes occurring in humanity's collective consciousness or shared psychic patterning. Seth was the first to mention this mass psychical event, calling it our period of "change" in his works. The term was first used in Elias sessions of the 1990s.

Solar Plexus chakra route – The solar plexus chakra center is concerned with processing psycho-electric data that relates to feelings and emotions.

State/s of being – A state of being describes a condition our consciousness is experiencing. There are two primary states of being from which other states derive, these are:

Being in **Divine Love** – meaning that our mind's **vibrational signature** is in vibrational alignment with this vital force steering all expressions of **Consciousness**.

Being in a state of fear – meaning that our vibrational signature is *not* in alignment with Divine Love—also referred to as being in a "state of resistance."

We often confuse states of being with **feelings**. Feelings are energy signals sent to your **conscious-mind** but by their nature *do not last*. States of being can last for a considerable time. Feeling happy, for example, is precisely that: a feeling that will fade, as it is not a state of being. Contentment, on the other hand, is an example of a state of being which generates feelings of happiness.

Subconscious/Subconscious area – The subconscious is an *area* within **Consciousness**. *Our* subconscious is an area within our mind that can provide us access to this area within Consciousness. It is a way station or bridge between the subjective (spiritual) and objective (physical) realms, a "place" where our inner self can communicate and interact with our physical self (**ego-self** and **personality**).

Throat chakra – This energy center processes information relating to our interactions with others—which includes all inorganic or organic *others*.

Vibrational signature – Your vibrational signature is the primal tone of your overall Self's identity.

"You create your own reality" – This term first appeared in *The*

[78]

Nature of Personal Reality: A Seth Book, authored by Jane Roberts in 1974. The "you" refers to your multidimensional Self—that is, the entirety of your being within Consciousness. The book explains how we can access our subconscious and begin to consciously express our multidimensional power.

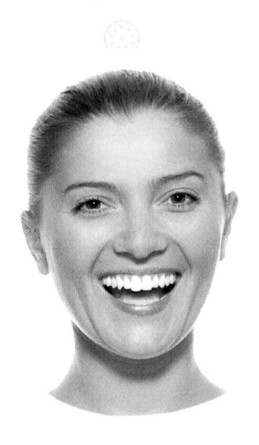

About the Author & Note to Reader

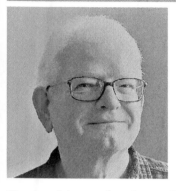

Chris W.E. Johnson

Chris began his study of channeled metaphysical literature following a personal life crisis in 1988. Studies of the Seth material (authored by Jane Roberts) awakened a passion for psychology and by 1998 he had earned a Master's Degree in Occupational and Organizational Psychology from the University of Surrey. During his academic studies he developed an in-depth knowledge of a variety of metaphysical offerings relating to the spiritual and psychological aspects to the "Self." He is considered a leading UK expert on Seth's teachings.

Since 2000, he's run *Counselling for your Self,* a complementary therapeutic practice that adopts an integral approach in combining his academic knowledge of psychotherapy with alternative procedures such as Energy Psychology techniques and guided meditation. Following his training under Dr. Brian Weiss in 2007, he added Past Life Regression Therapy to his therapeutic arsenal.

Chris has presented internationally on his findings and interpretations of metaphysical knowledge since 2003. He developed a series of experiential workshops, first rolled out in the autumn of 2009, specifically designed to bring others a fuller appreciation of their "Self" and their intentional leanings. He became a member of the Scientific and Medical Network in 2011.

From the Author:
I am deeply grateful and appreciative of your interest in this book. I

[80]

sincerely hope that its content has been as revelatory, encouraging, and Self-satisfying as I found it to be while creating it. If you have a few moments, I would be grateful if you would add a review to your favorite online site by way of feedback.

Feelings Explained: Emotions Tamed is a reworked extraction from the first edition of *It's About You! Know Your Self,* published in June 2013 by O-Books. *Know Your Self* is the first book in the *It's About You!* trilogy.

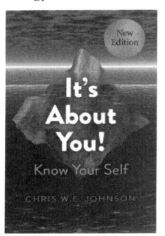

The trilogy is a synthesis of the profound knowledge found in metaphysical, philosophical and scientific literature about the "Self," and how we go about creating our physical experiences.

A re-edited and updated New Edition of *It's About You! Know Your Self* was released by O-Books on Jan 31st, 2020. Book II, *Free Your Self,* is still in writing as of December 2019.

Do visit my website for news of Book II, my other offerings, blog posts, and to sign up for my newsletter.

cwejohnson.com

Also by Chris W.E. Johnson:

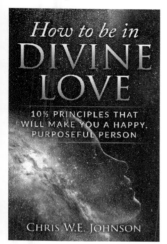

How to be in DIVINE LOVE

10% PRINCIPLES THAT WILL MAKE YOU A HAPPY, PURPOSEFUL PERSON

CHRIS W.E. JOHNSON

Book I in the 'Being Human' series.

This book will help you to come to terms with our collective shift in consciousness and lay the foundations for you to ride the "Shift."

You will learn of the absolute undistorted spiritual principles that steer the creation of your life's reality. These "natural" principles are not a set of laws or commandments from on high; they are a purified set of mental behavioral guidelines—unadulterated by institutional dogma. They are the human psyche's translation of the universal force behind all creation—the vitality of Divine Love.

The natural principles are the human psyche's translation of how the universe works—how Consciousness endeavors to know itself through its creation of the human species—and thus, through you. They are the fundamental principles by which Divine Love can operate through you—through your unique individualized expression of Consciousness. They exist for you to construct a necessary mental inclination, a magical mind-set, which will enable you to create the experiences you prefer from life.

Divine Love is a state of being. That is, you can *be* in Divine Love—through observing the natural principles for as much as you can throughout your life.

A review from the first edition:

"A Wonderful Guide for Those Who are Feeling a Little Lost These Days!"

[82]

We live in a time when many people (and especially the younger folks) are finding the moral and ethical anchors being cut away. It's fine to scrutinize what drives our behavior, but currently it seems we have little to guide us other than rampant media messages of simply taking care of yourself and ignoring others. This book is a great guide of 10 principles that can help provide a way out of the collective morass and initiate thought-provoking concepts on defining who we want to be. I recommend this for many who are searching for their personal guidance in a spiritual setting and to be effective in day-to-day relationships."- David Barnett, BA, BS, MS.

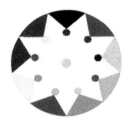

Printed in Great Britain
by Amazon